See.

Ruth Thomson

Photographs by Peter Millard

Contents

Look at your eyes	2
Eye see	4
Shut eye	6
Out of sight	8
Pupil power	10
One eye or two?	12
Moving together	14
Near and far	16
Seeing in colour	18
What can you see?	20
Fooling your eyes	22
Index	24

W

FRANKLIN WATTS

LONDON • NEW YORK • SYDNEY

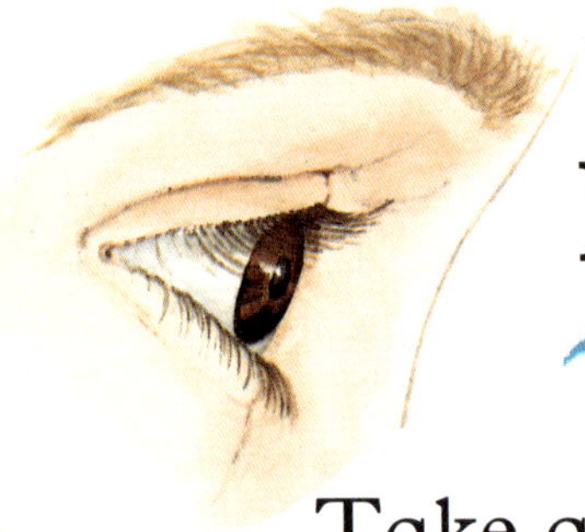

Look at your eyes

Take a look at your eyes in a mirror.
Notice how they are set back well
into your face.
They are protected by a bony socket.
Feel the bones with your fingers.

The coloured circle is called the iris.
The black spot in the middle of it
is a hole, called the pupil.
Your pupils let light into your eyes.

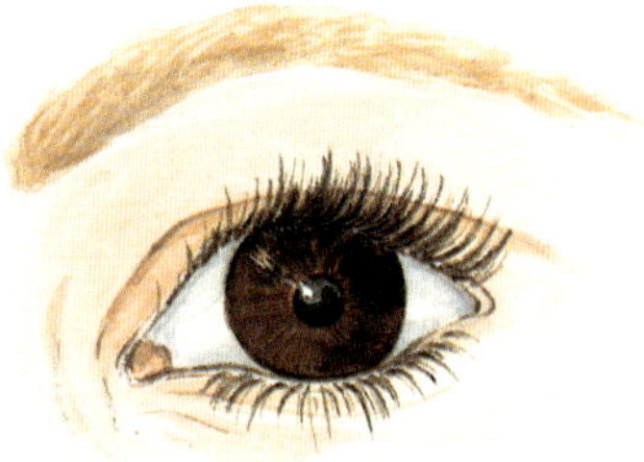

Your eyelids protect your eyes
and keep them moist.
Every time you blink, your eyelids
spread tears over your eyes.
Your eyelashes stop dust and dirt
from brushing against your eyes.

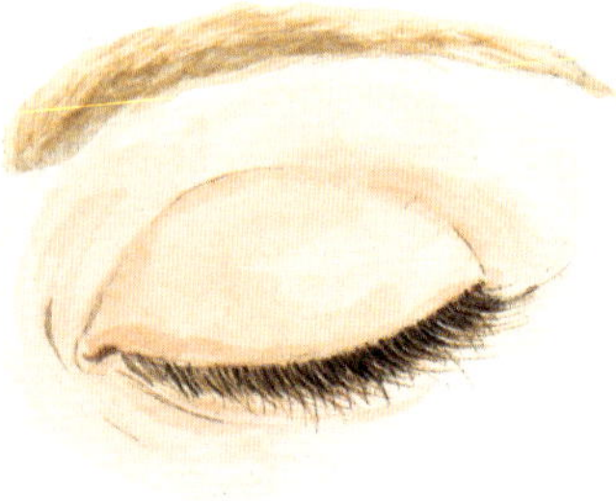

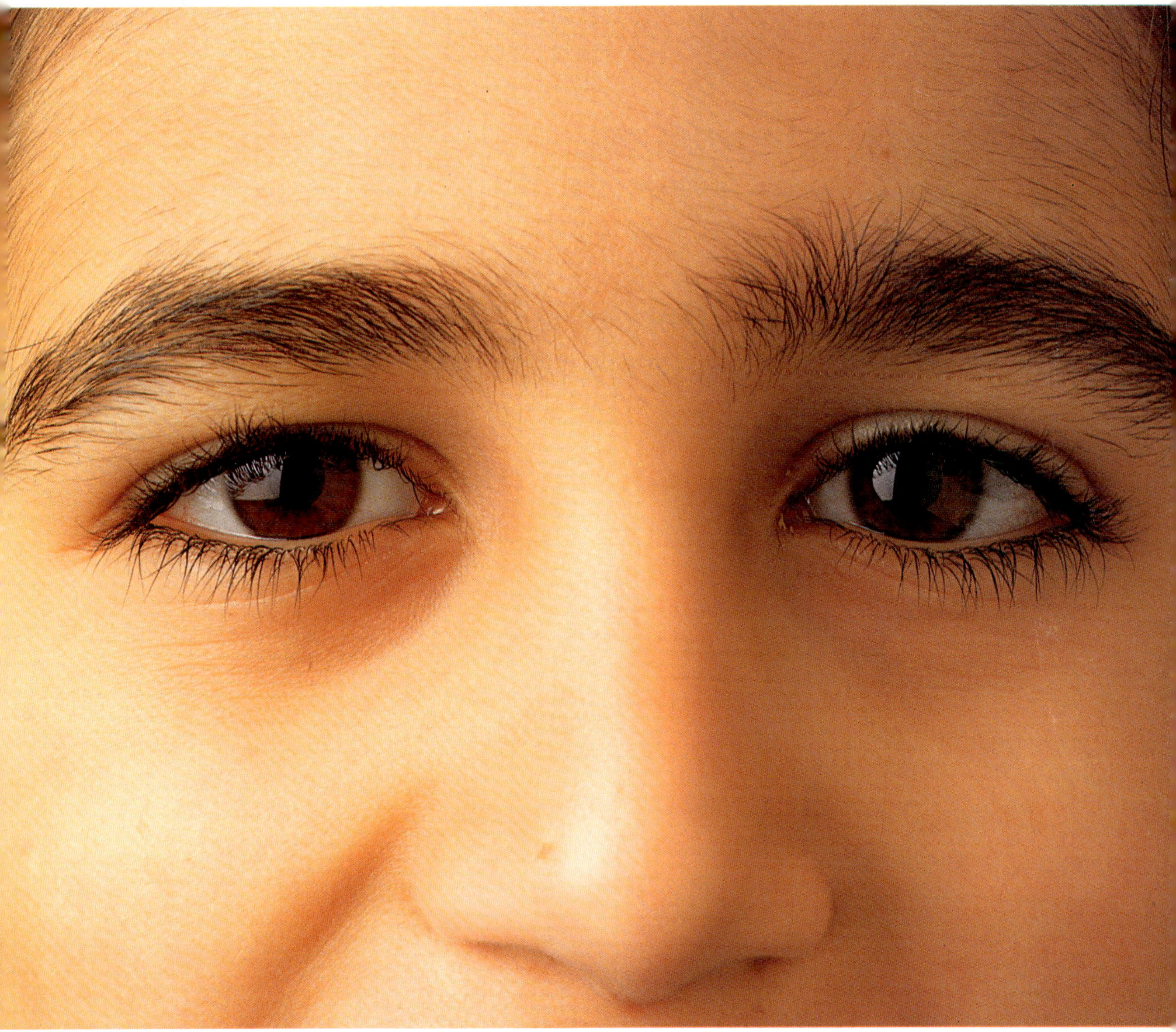

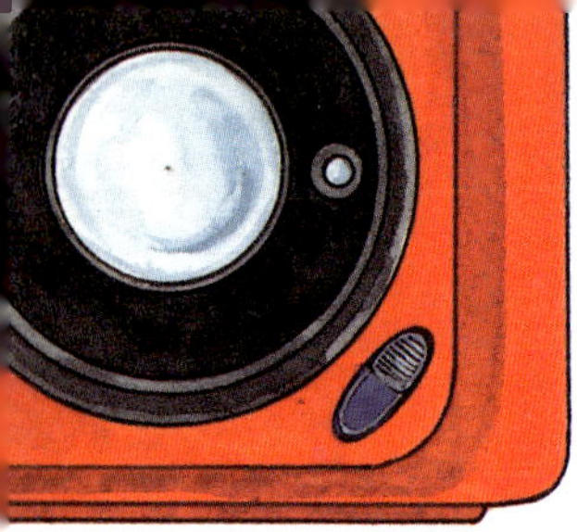

Eye see

Each eye has a lens.
It works like a lens in a camera.
It lets in light from everything
you see around you.

The lens bends the light.
Upside-down pictures are formed
on the lining at the back of the eye.
This lining is called the retina.

The retina sends signals to the brain
about the light pattern of the pictures.
The brain sorts out the signals
and works out what you are seeing.

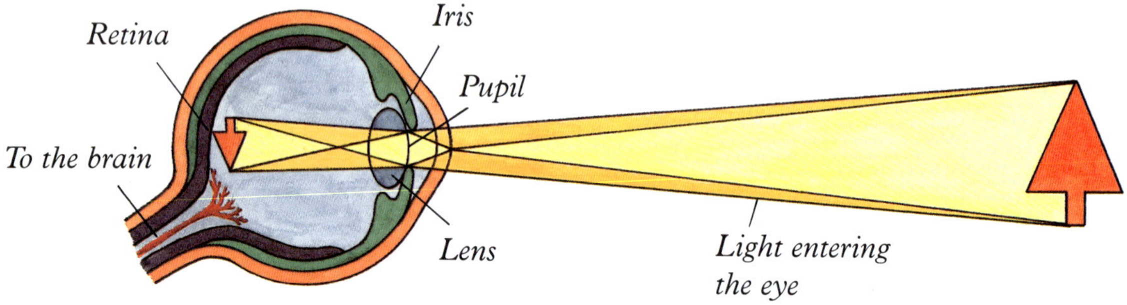

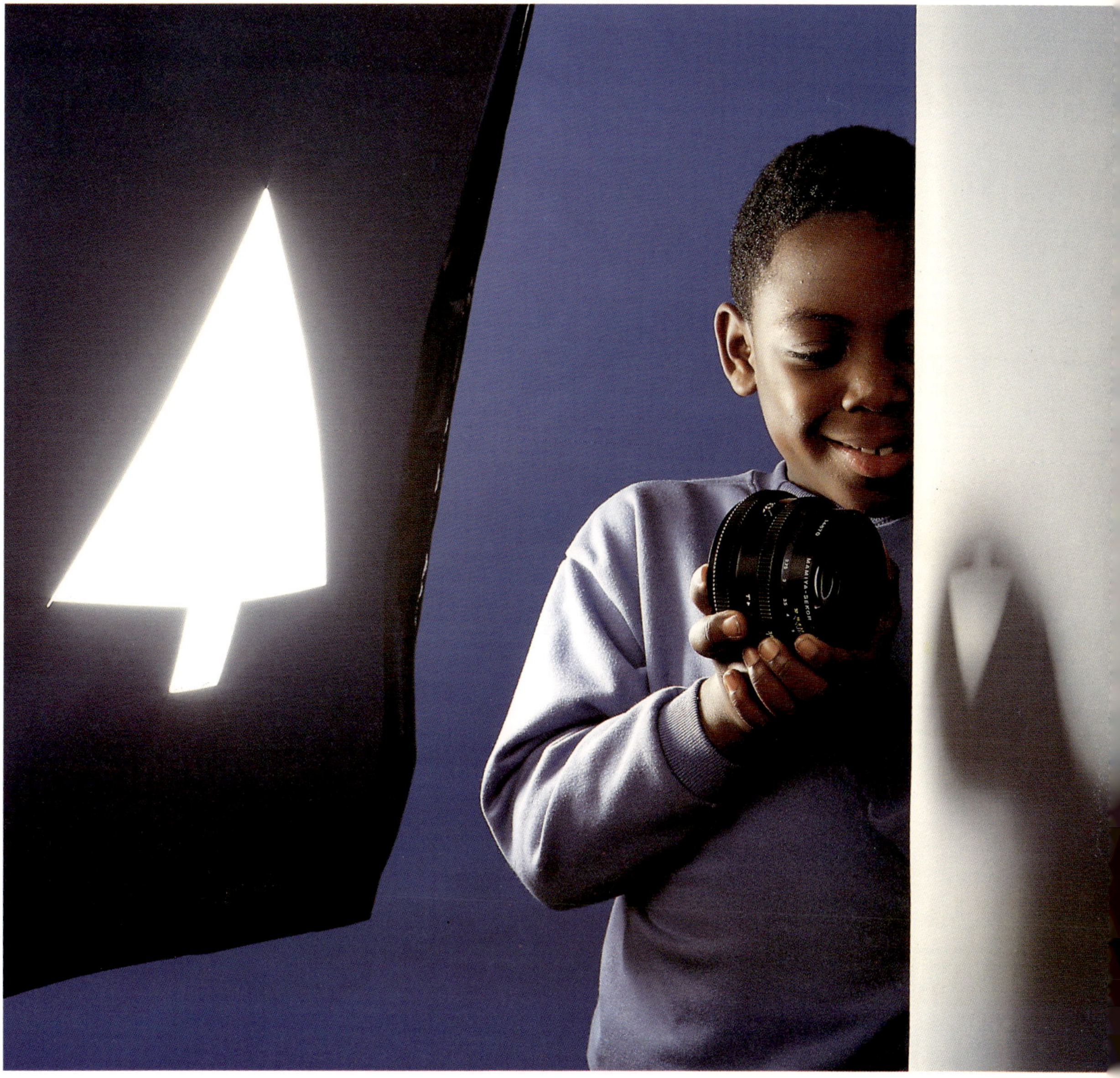

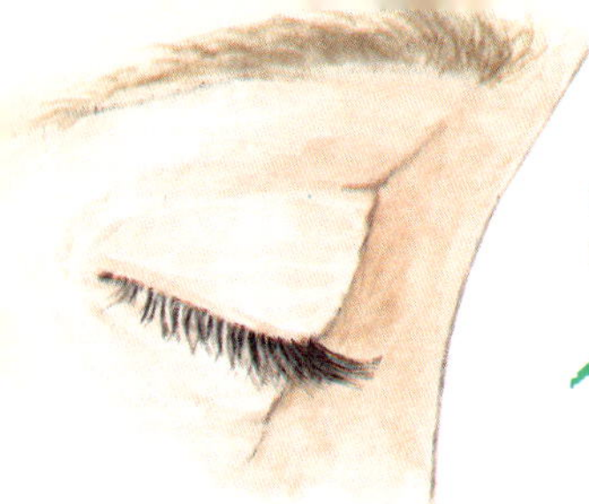

Shut eye

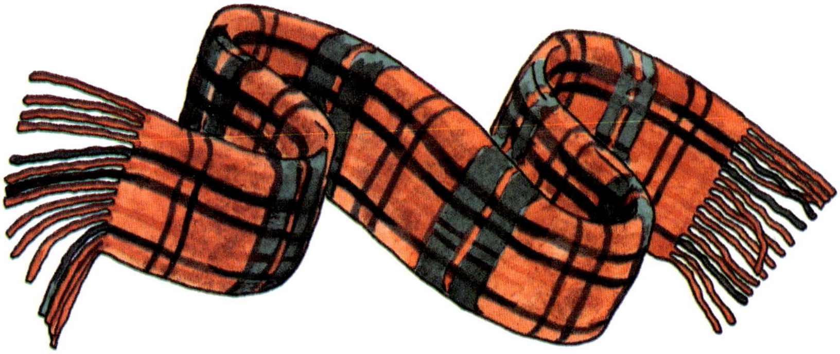

Get ready

✔Blindfold

...Get set

Blindfold a friend in the middle of a room.
Turn her around once or twice.
Stand by the door and clap your hands.
Ask your friend to walk to the door.

Go!

Watch how your friend moves.
What senses does she use to help her?
How easily can she reach you
if you stop clapping?

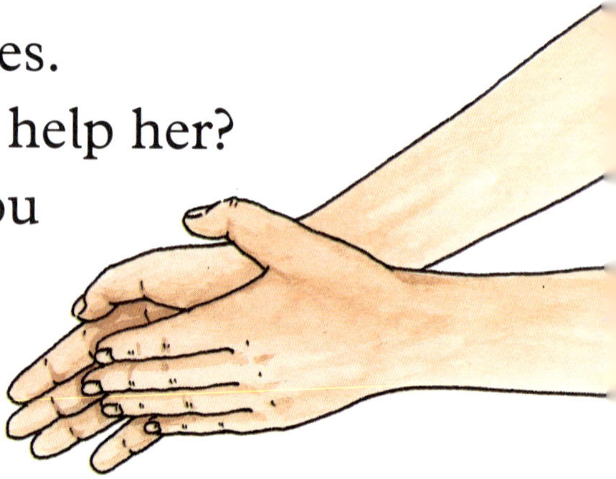

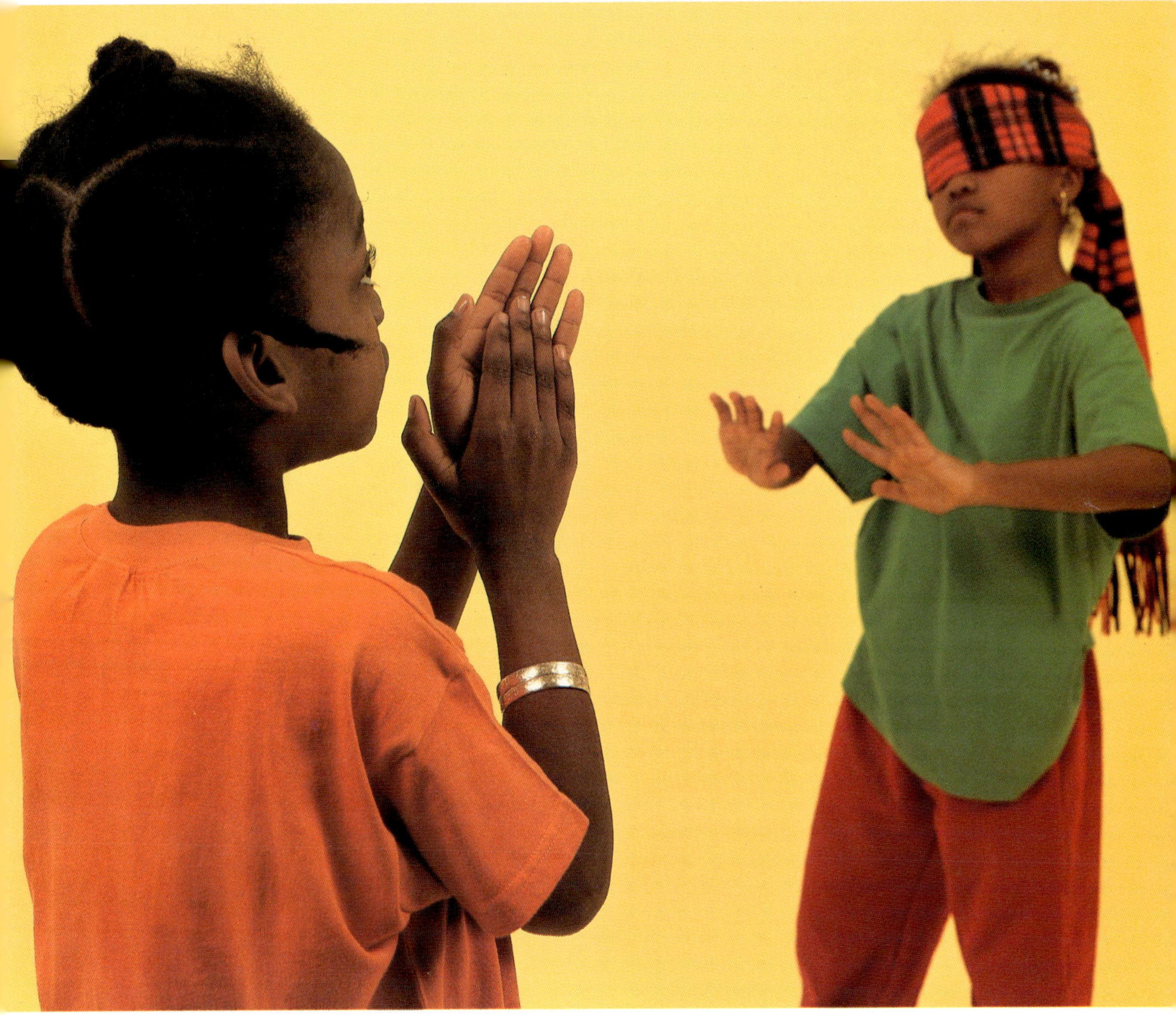

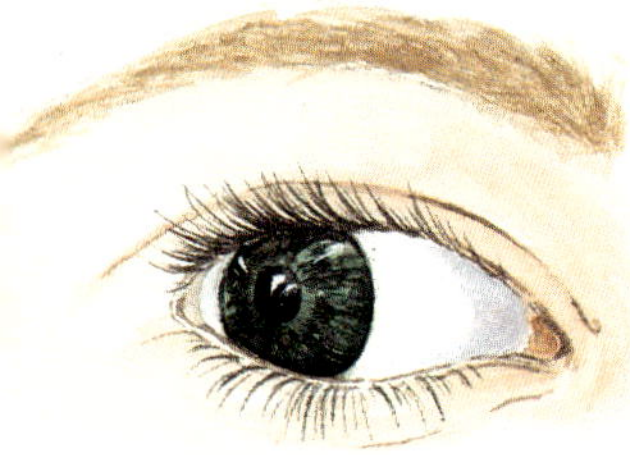

Out of sight

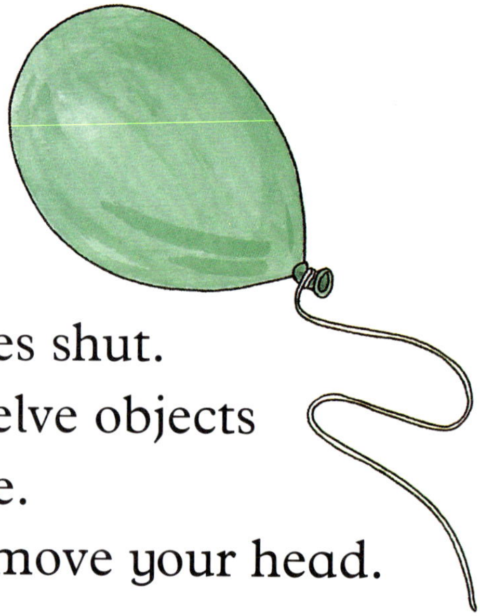

Get ready

✔ 12 different small objects

...Get set

Sit on the floor with your eyes shut.
Ask a friend to space the twelve objects evenly around you in a circle.
Open your eyes, but do not move your head.

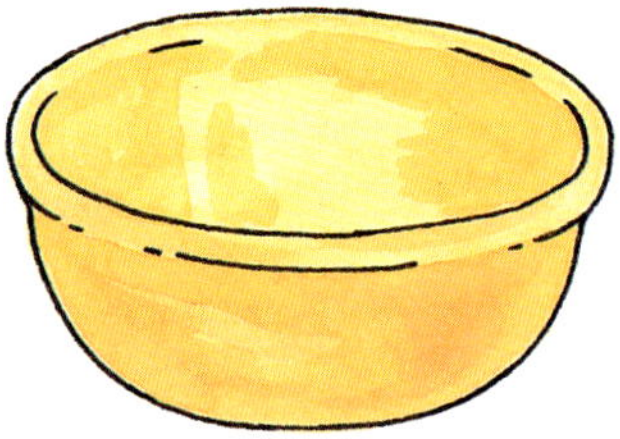

Go!

How many things can you see?
How many more can you see if you turn your head from side to side?
Can you see everything if you twist your head?

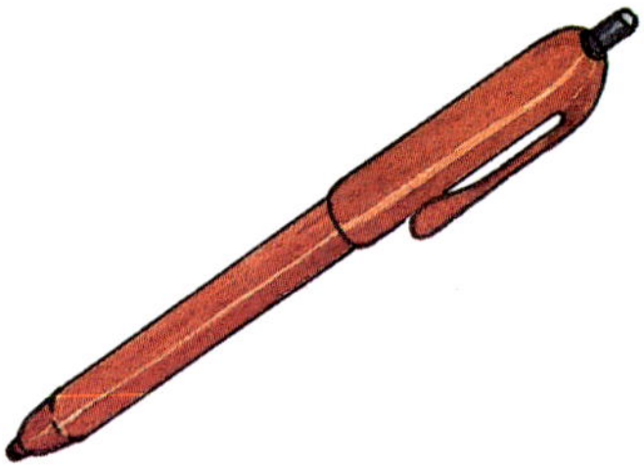

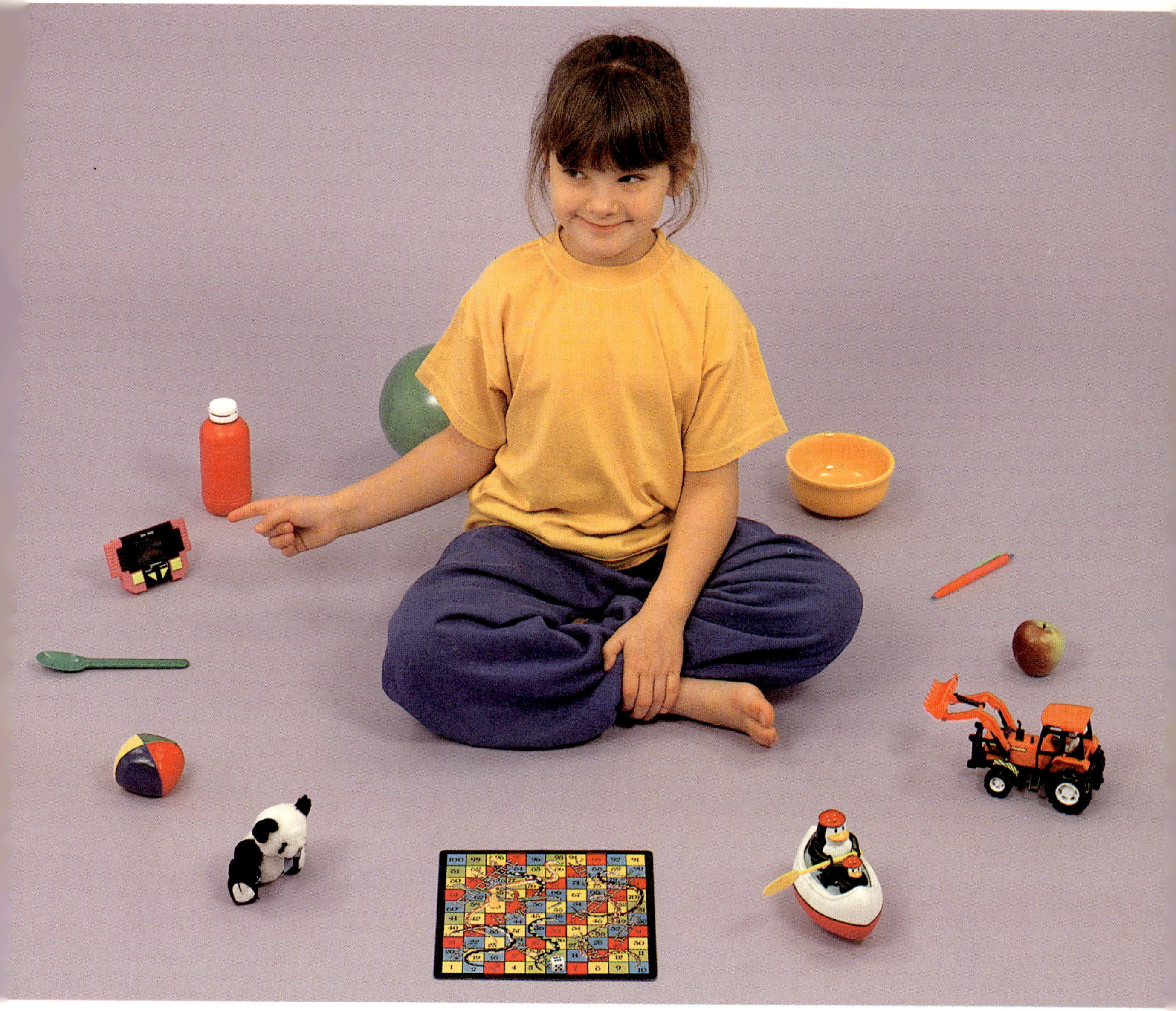

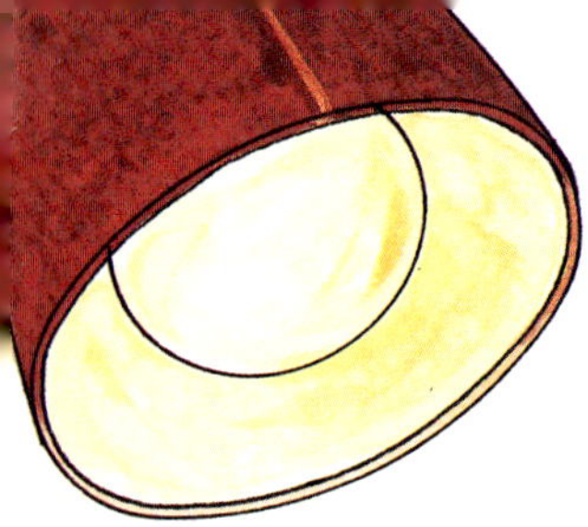

Pupil power

Get ready

✔Lamp ✔Mirror

...Get set

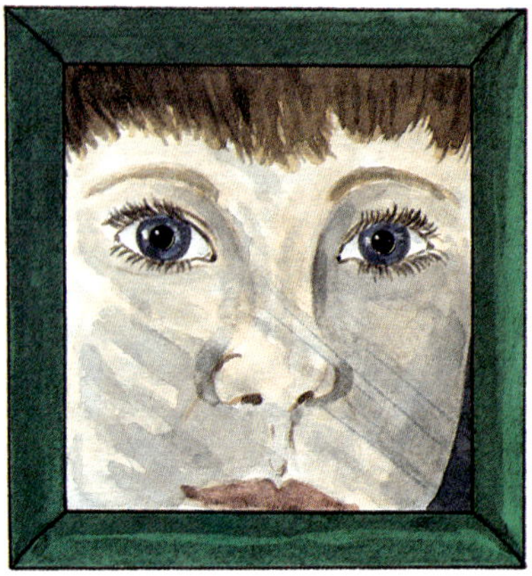

Look at your pupils
in a mirror
in a darkened room.
Notice their size.
Then turn on a lamp.

Go!

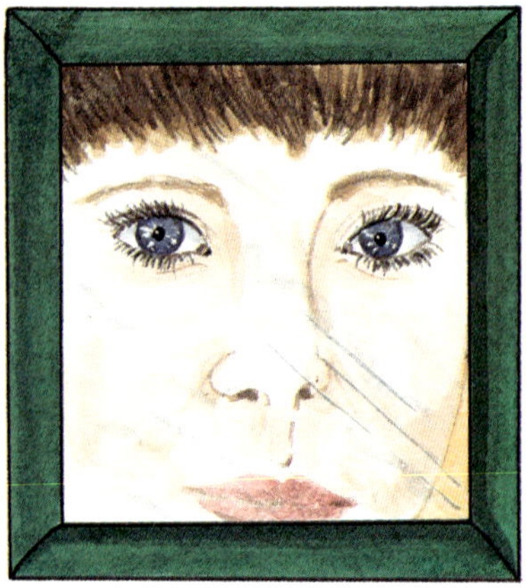

What happens
to your pupils now?
Why do you think
they change?

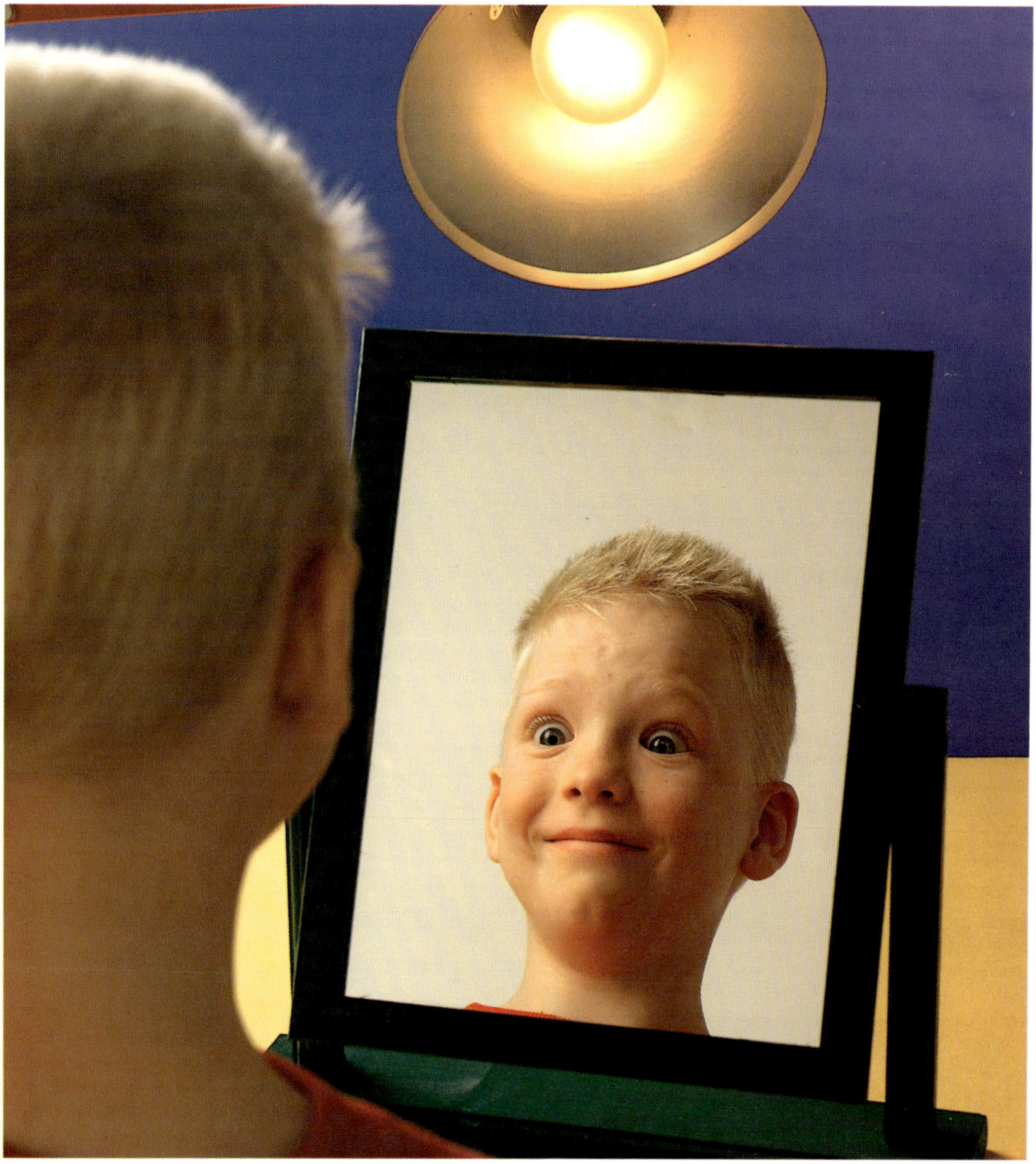

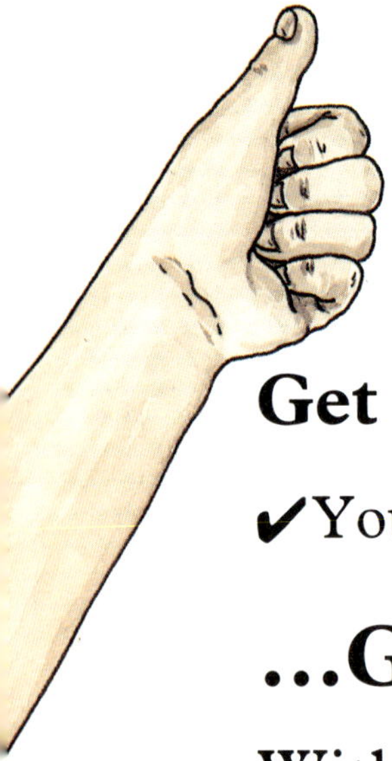

One eye or two?

Get ready

✔Your thumb

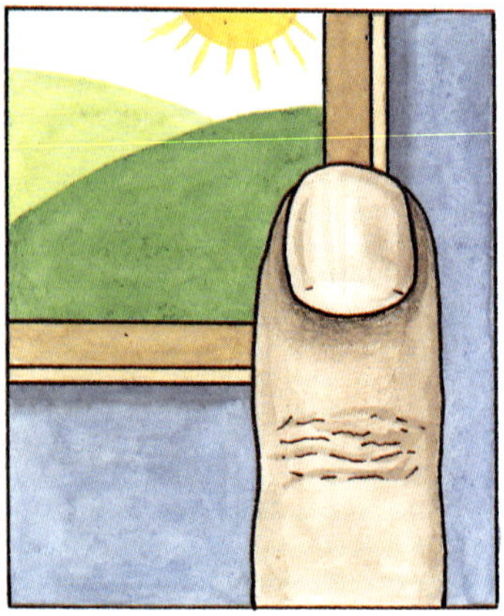

...Get set

With one eye closed, hold up
a thumb at arm's length.
Line it up with the upright edge
of a door or a picture.
Open your closed eye.
Close the other eye.

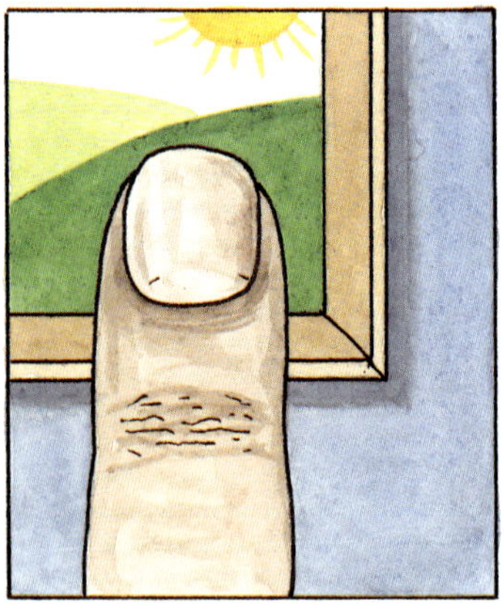

Go!

What happens to your thumb?

Each eye sees a separate picture.
Your brain puts the two pictures together.
This helps you to work out how far away
things are and makes them look solid.

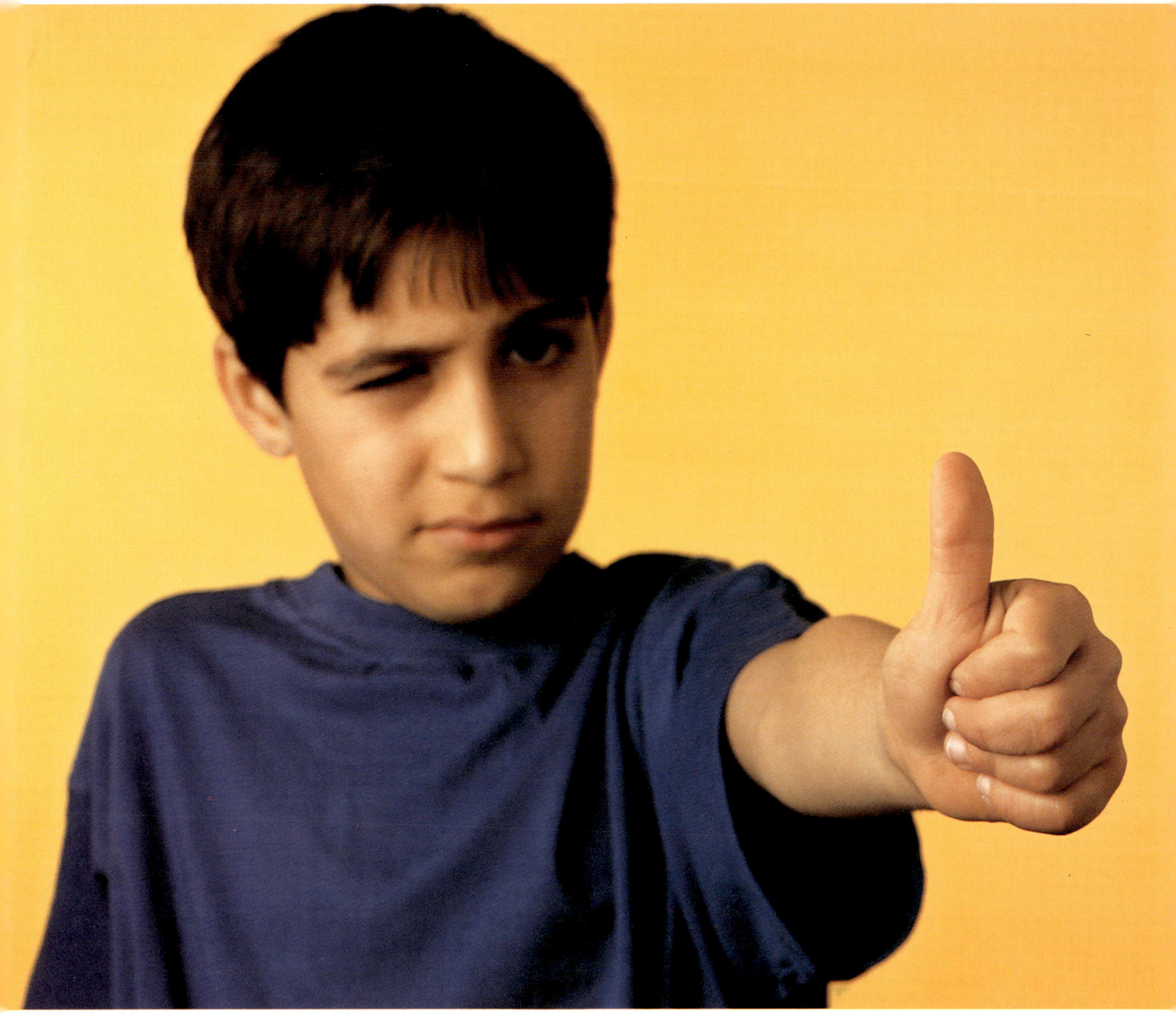

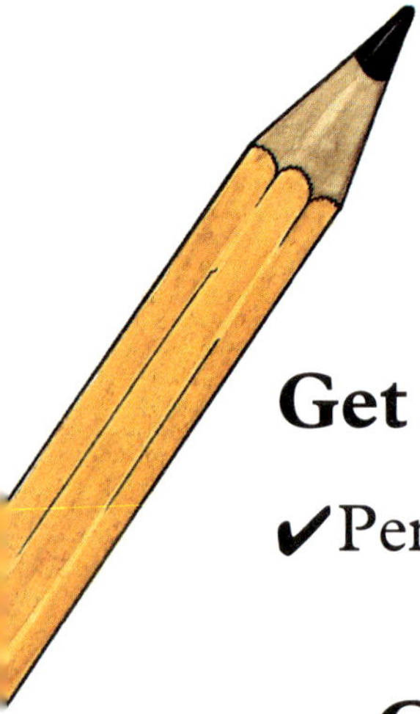

Moving together

Get ready

✔Pencil

...Get set

Hold a pencil about 30 cm
away from your face.
Move it to the left
and then to the right.
Bring it close to your nose.

Go!

Ask a friend to watch your eyes.
Do both eyes move separately or together?
What happens when they look
at something very close?

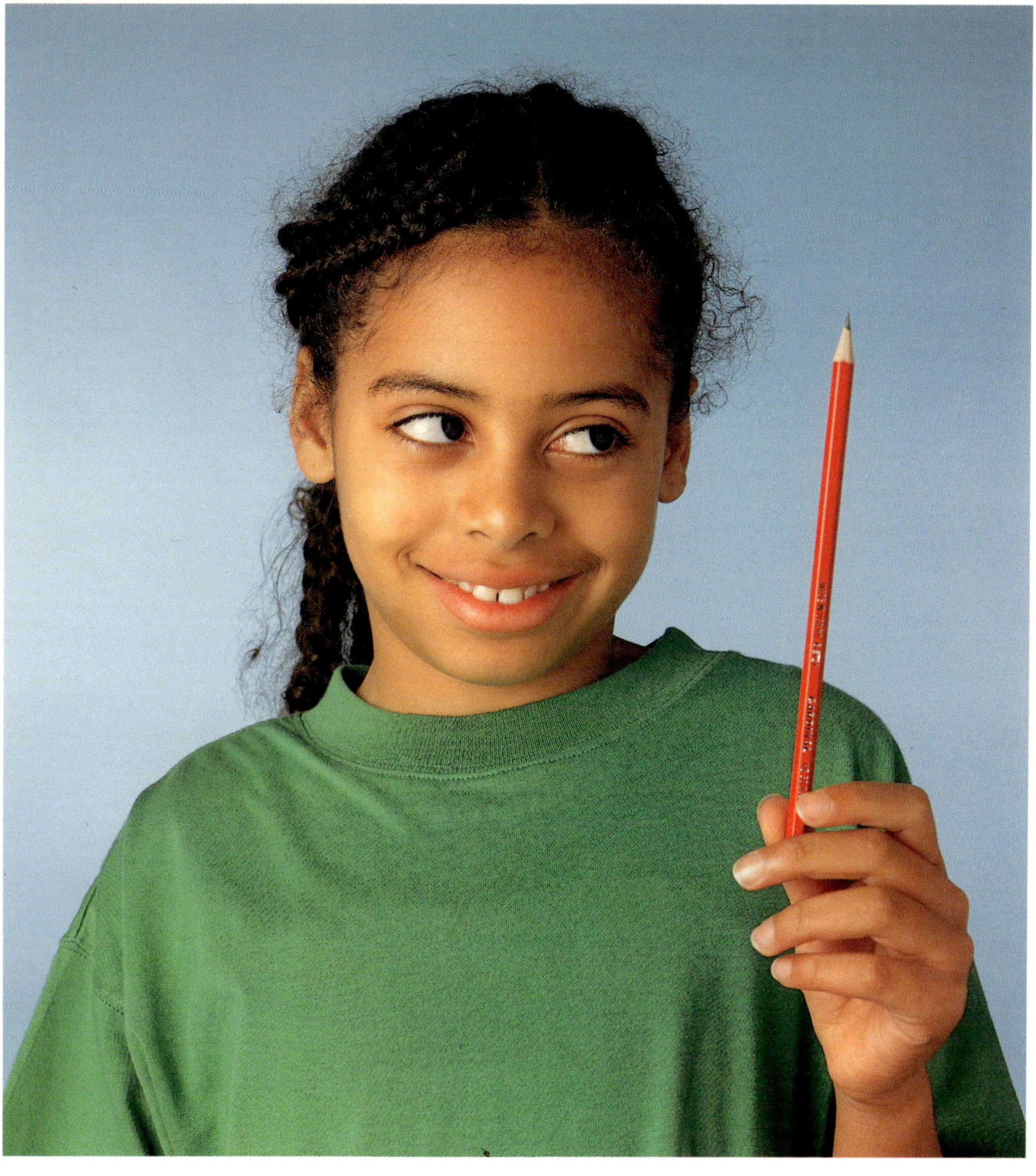

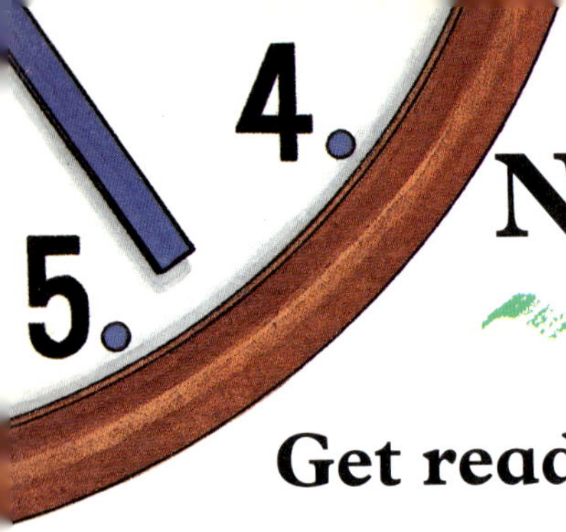

Near and far

Get ready

✔Book ✔Clock or picture

...Get set

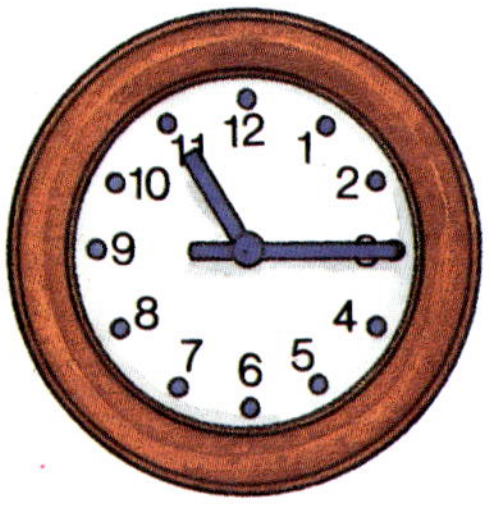

Read some words in a book.
Quickly look up at a clock
or a picture on the wall.
Then look back at the book.

Go!

What do you notice?

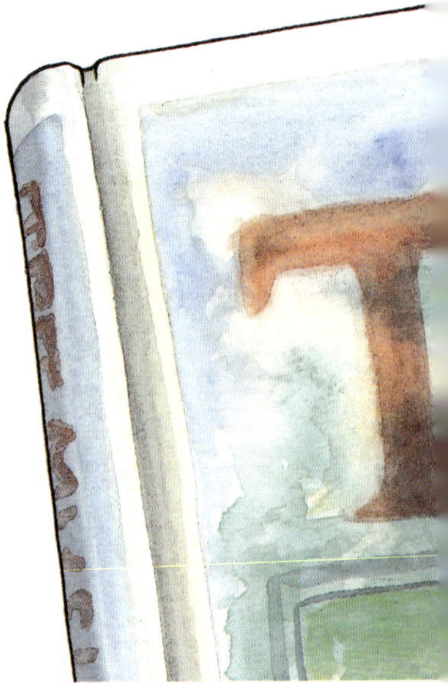

Your eyes can only focus clearly
on one thing at a time.
This is why things look blurred
when you shift your gaze.

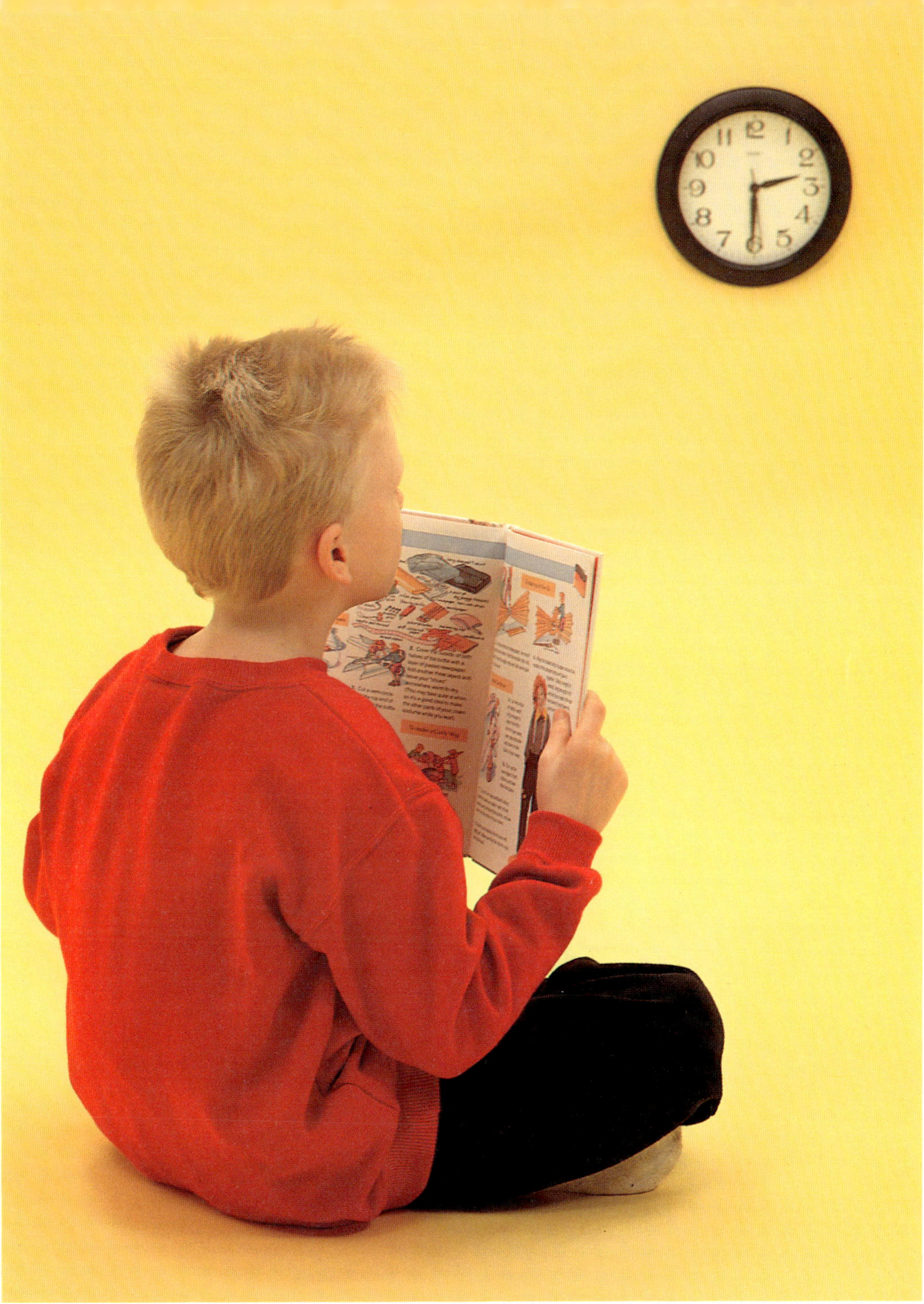

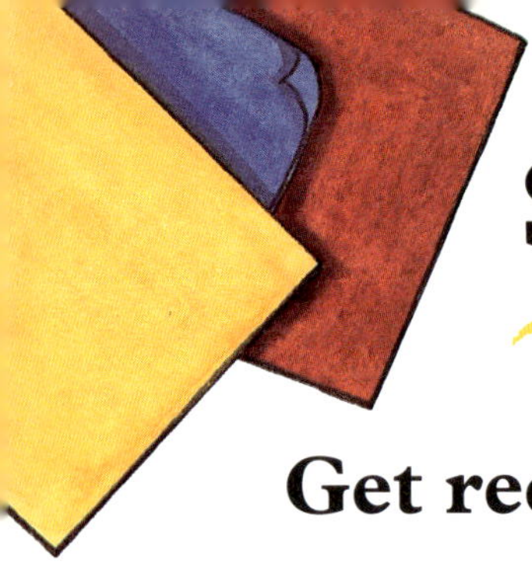

Seeing in colour

Get ready

✔Sheets of different coloured paper
(at least two sheets of each colour)

...Get set

Close the curtains or make a dark corner with a blanket and some chairs.
Lay out the sheets of paper.
Try to match sheets of the same colour.

Go!

Are paler shades or bright ones easier to match?
What difference does it make when you try matching the sheets in bright light?

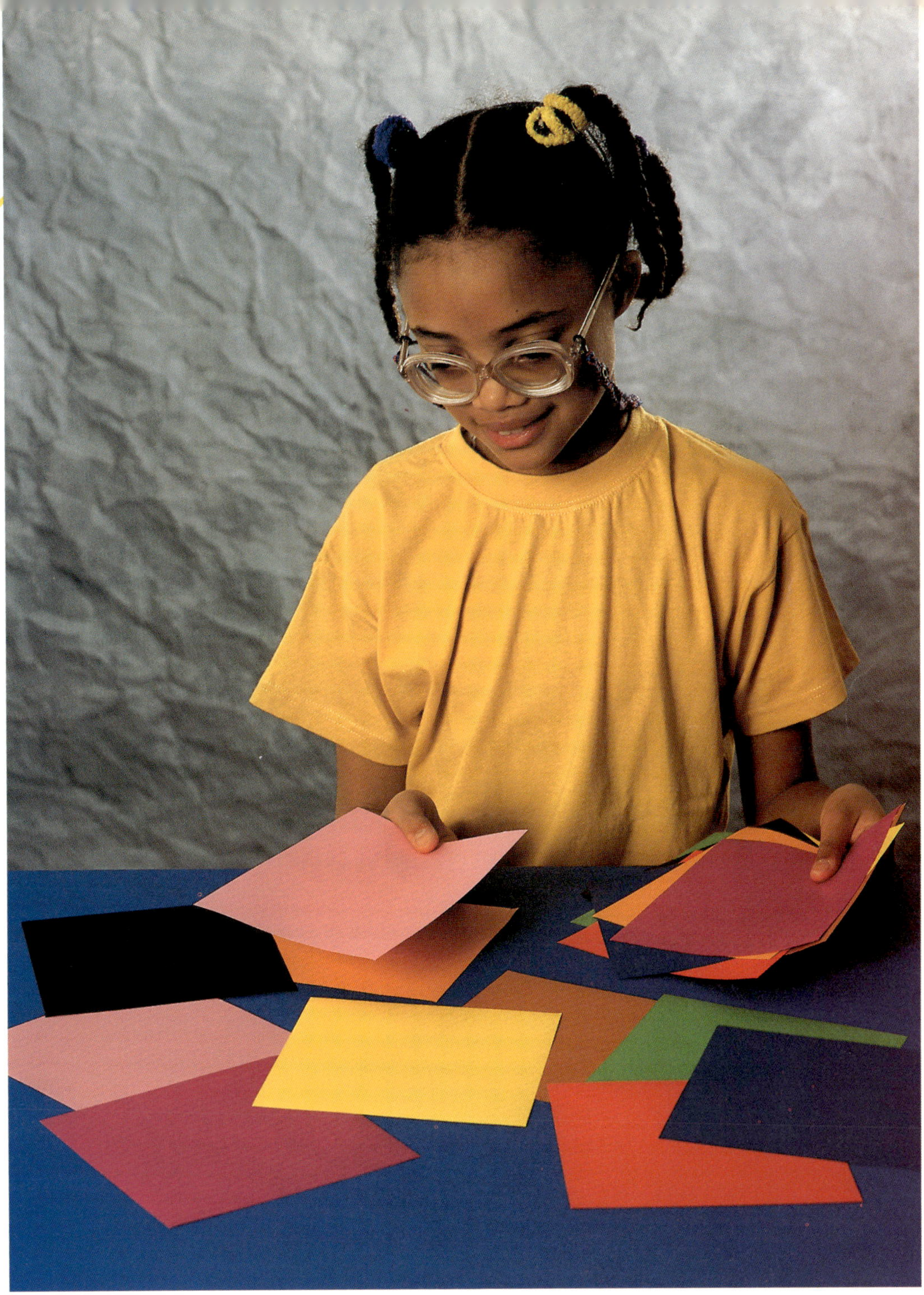

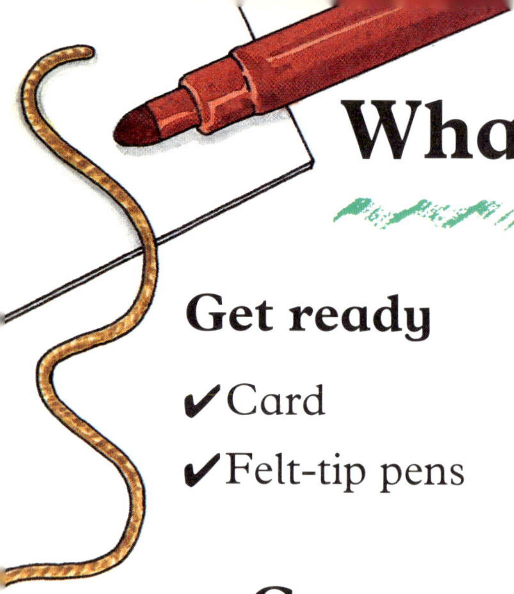

What can you see?

Get ready

✔Card ✔Cup ✔Pencil
✔Felt-tip pens ✔Scissors ✔String

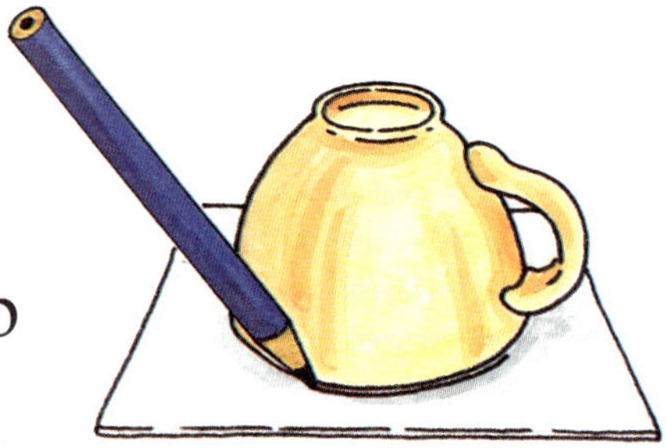

...Get set

Make a card circle, using a cup to draw around, and cut it out. Draw and colour an animal on one side. Draw a cage, net or bowl on the other one. Thread a length of string through a hole on both sides of the circle and knot the ends

Go!

Twizzle the string.
What can you see?

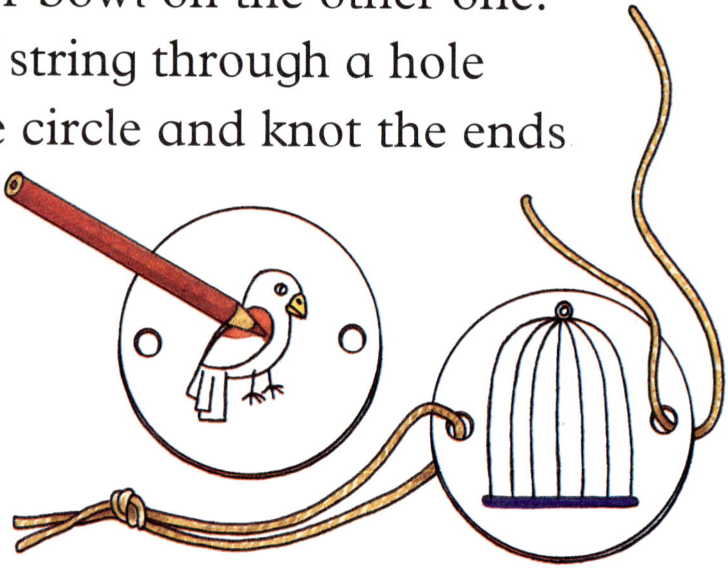

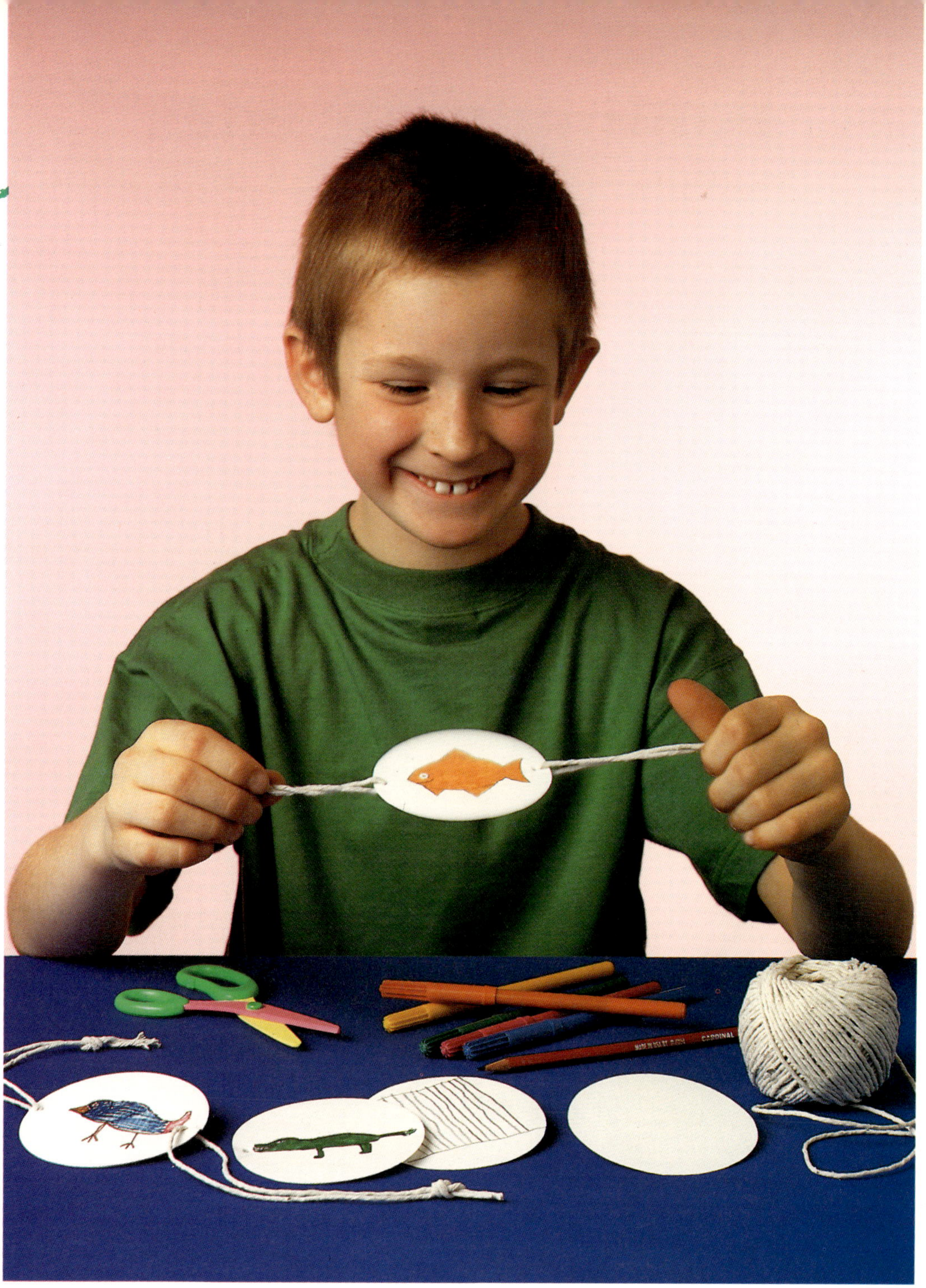

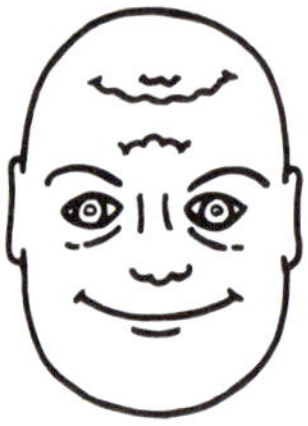

Fooling your eyes

Your eyes and brain can play tricks.

Look at the black squares. What can you see where the white lines cross?

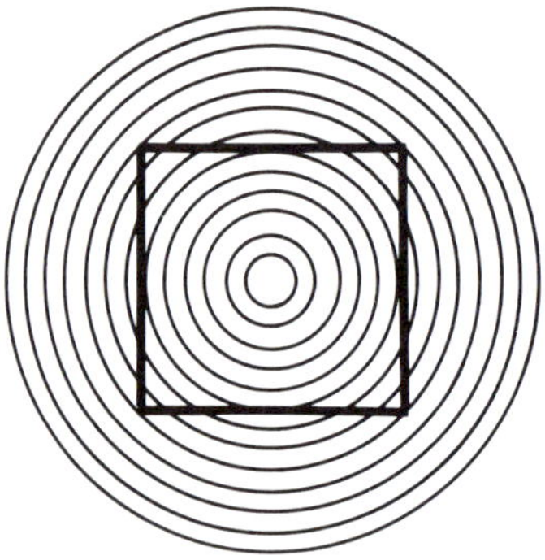

Is this square straight or bent? Check with a ruler.

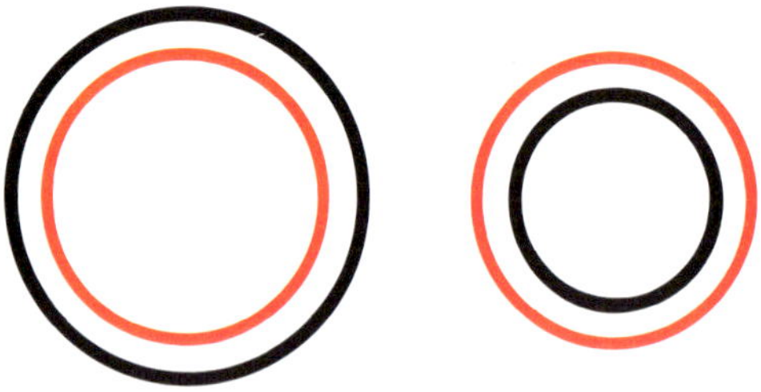

Which of the red circles is bigger? Measure them.

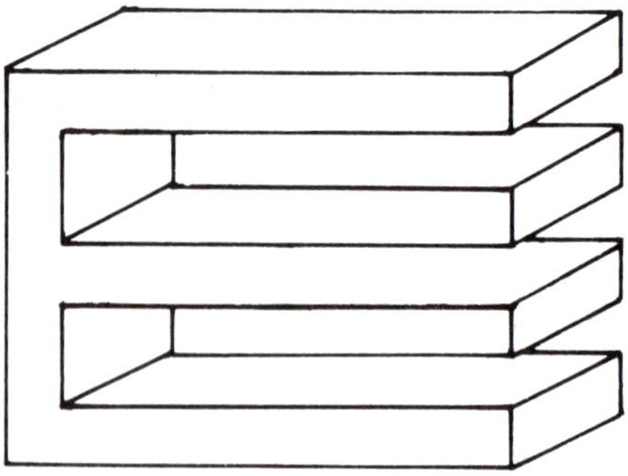

Does this shape have three or four arms?

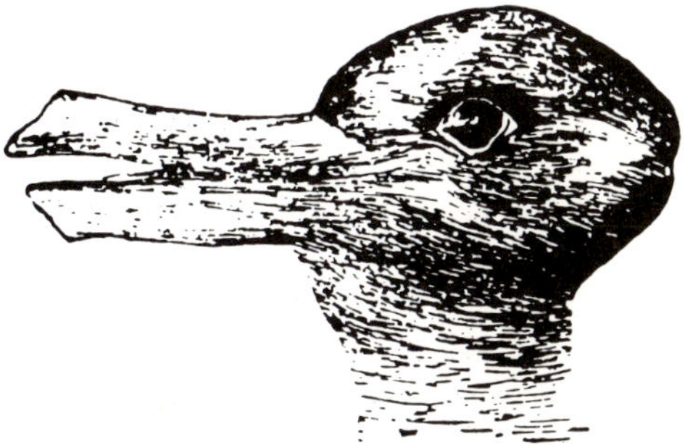

Is this a duck,
or is it a rabbit?

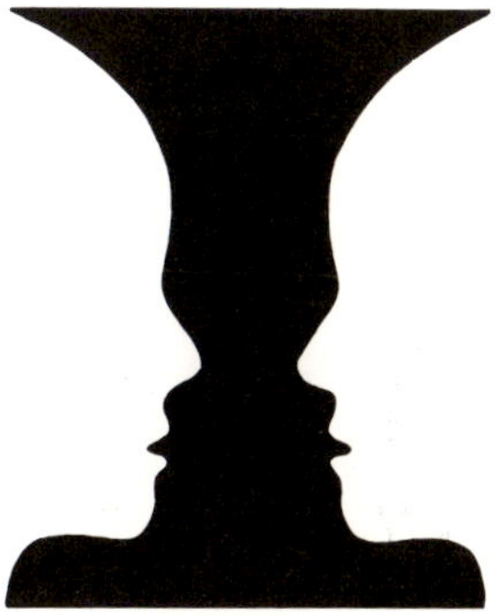

Can you see a vase
or two faces?

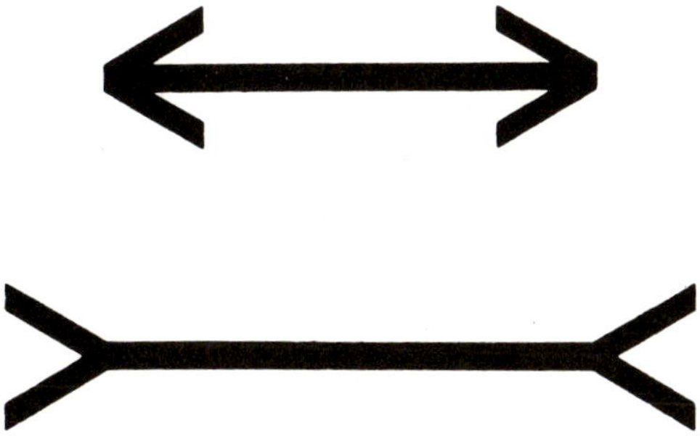

Which arrow is longer?
Measure them and see.

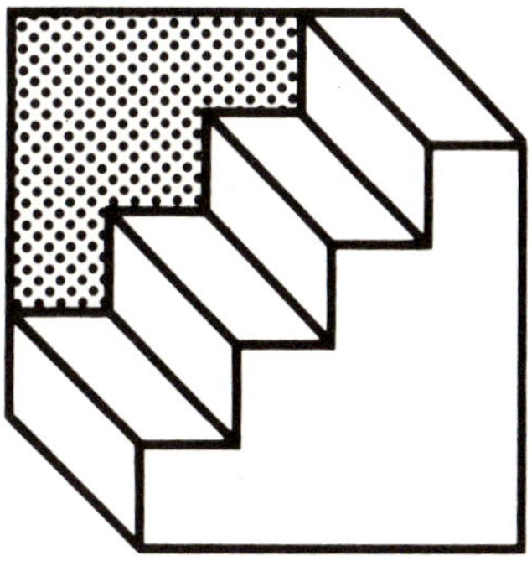

Are you next to the stairs
or underneath them?

Index

Words that appear in *italics* decribe the ideas behind the activities.

blindfold 6
blink 2
book 16
brain 4, 12
bright light 10, 18

clock 16
coloured paper 18

dark room 10, 18

eye 2, 4, 6, 12, 14
eyelashes 2
eyelids 2

felp-tip pens 20

fooling your eyes 22–23

how you see 4

iris 2

lamp 10
lens 4

mirror 2, 10

pencil 14, 20
picture 12, 16

pupil 2, 10

reading 16
retina 4

seeing
behind you 8
blurred 16
colours 18
in the dark 10, 18
socket 2
string 20

tears 2
thumb 12

using both eyes 12

Acknowledgments:
The author and publisher would like to thank the pupils of Kenmont Primary School, London, for their participation in the photographs of this book.

Paperback edition 1996

Franklin Watts
96 Leonard Street
London EC2A 4RH

Franklin Watts Australia
14 Mars Road
Lane Cove
NSW 2066

UK ISBN 0 7496 1675 X (hardback)
0 7496 2639 9 (paperback)

Series Editor: Pippa Pollard
Editor: Annabel Martin
Design: Ruth Levy
Cover design: Nina Kingsbury
Artwork: Ruth Levy

A CIP catalogue record for this book is available from the British Library

Dewey Decimal Classification 612.8

Printed in Malaysia